Strength Training for Beginners

A Guide to Weight Lifting and Weight Training

By: Robert Young

9781631871719

I0414091

PUBLISHER'S NOTES

Disclaimer – Speedy Publishing, LLC

This publication is intended to provide helpful and informative material. It is not intended to diagnose, treat, cure, or prevent any health problem or condition, nor is intended to replace the advice of a physician. No action should be taken solely on the contents of this book. Always consult your physician or qualified healthcare professional on any matters regarding your health and before adopting any suggestions in this book or drawing inferences from it.

The author and publisher specifically disclaim all responsibility for any liability, loss or risk, personal or otherwise, which is incurred as a consequence, directly or indirectly, from the use or application of any contents of this book.

Any and all product names referenced within this book are the trademarks of their respective owners. None of these owners have sponsored, authorized, endorsed, or approved this book.

Always read all information provided by the manufacturers' product labels before using their products. The author and publisher are not responsible for claims made by manufacturers.

This book was originally printed before 2014. This is an adapted reprint by Speedy Publishing LLC with newly updated content designed to help readers with much more accurate and timely information and data.

Speedy Publishing, LLC©2014

40 E. Main Street #1156

Newark, Delaware

19711

Contact Us: 1-888-248-4521

Website: http://www.speedypublishing.com

REPRINTED Paperback Edition: ISBN: 9781631871719

Manufactured in the United States of America

DEDICATION

This book is dedicated to those who view their body as a temple. Nothing is wrong with taking pride in who you are and taking care of your body. Weightlifting simply helps to enhance the way the body looks. It is great exercise as well!

TABLE OF CONTENTS

Robert Young

INTRODUCTION - WHY LIFT WEIGHTS?

Whether you call it weightlifting, pumping iron, or bodybuilding - lifting weights both light and heavy has long been a great way to get in shape and stay in shape. Weightlifting or weight training has many health benefits for both men and women. There are weightlifting and weight-training routines appropriate for men, woman, even children of any age, any size, and any body type. If you want to build muscle mass, increase stamina, improve cardiac function, even stave off the symptoms of osteoporosis - you can accomplish all of that and so much more by adding a good weight training routine to your regular workout.

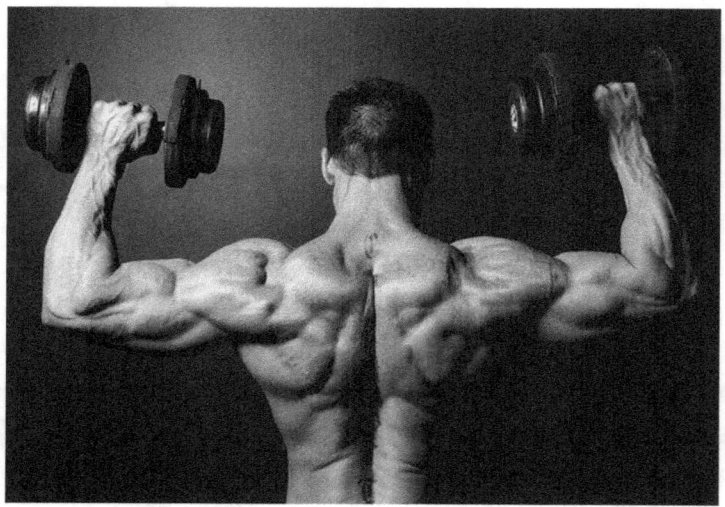

To get the most health benefit out of lifting weights, you need to combine your weight training with other exercise. If you are not already doing some kind of aerobic or cardio workout every day you must do this in addition to weight lifting. It is not healthy to just begin to lift weights without a proper warm up; of course before starting any workout routine check with your doctor. Prior to starting your weight lifting workout you need to "get the blood moving" and your muscles primed for some heavy lifting.

Just before hitting the weights do a good ten minutes on a bicycle, take a short jog, or jump rope. Do a few legs and arm stretch as well. The key to successful weight training involves what are called repetitions. In lifting it is not so important how much you lift, but how many times you can lift the weight. A proper weight lifting routine will be designed to work out all of the major muscle groups of the body, which include: The Shoulders, Neck and Back, Biceps, Triceps, Quadriceps Chest, Abs, Hamstrings, Calves, and of course the Gluteus.

The next question on your mind is likely to be "should I use free weights or machines?" and "how much weight should I work out with?" You can use free weights or machines or maybe a little of both. If you are working out in a gym, of course they will have both and will likely be able to recommend a "circuit" of weight lifting exercises for you. If you intend to lift weights in the home, it all depends on your budget and physical space to determine if you want to buy a "Home Gym" type resistance trainer such as Bow flex - or a good set of free weights and barbells - or both.

Weight machines are great for beginners because they have been designed to work a specific muscle or muscle group, and will insure that you are seated or standing in the right position to target that group when you lift. Free weights are the traditional barbells and dumbbells that have been around for centuries, and they work great. In fact, some would argue that once you learn how to use them properly, you get a better workout than machines because it is only the force of your muscles and your ability to balance the weight that keeps the weight and your muscles moving properly. There is no aid from the machine, so you are effectively using more muscle with free weights.

Lifting weights improves your strength and stamina. Lifting weights builds muscle and confidence, improves cardiovascular health and can actually help prevent other sports injuries. And lifting weights can help you lose extra pounds and keep them off - so what are you "weighting" for come on get pumping!

How does Weightlifting Increase Muscle Size?

We all know that lifting weights lead to bigger muscles, harder muscles, and more definition. But just how does weight lifting do that? What is the physiology of weight lifting?

Basically, weight lifting is a method of strength training. Lifting weights uses the force of gravity to oppose muscle contraction. Overcoming that opposition increases strength and builds muscle. The concept was simply and elegantly summed up by Hippocrates centuries ago – "That which is used develops, and that which is unused wastes away". He was correct – and his contemporaries while not sure of the anatomical science behind it, also understood the basic weight lifting and strength-training concept of progressive resistance. It's been said that ancient Greek wrestlers when training for the early Olympic Games carried a newborn calf on their back every day until it was grown. While that may not go over very well in your gym, the concept is sound. Weight lifting builds strength and muscle mass through progressive resistance. The reason our muscles grow and become stronger when we work out with weights is due to the body's response to injury. Muscle growth from weight lifting is basically a healing process. When we lift weights, we do (when done correctly) a small amount of micro trauma to our muscle tissue. The body's response to the trauma is to rebuild the weakened or torn muscle fibers, and in doing so build them even bigger and stronger than they were prior to the micro trauma so as to prevent a repeat of the injury. So that is how progressive resistance works in weight lifting and weight training.

We add more weight do more reps, and tear down more muscle fiber - the body keeps responding by healing the muscle eventually pushing the muscle to its ultimate limit, which is genetically determined.

Professional power lifters, other athletes, and experienced weightlifters will use this concept when training or working with weights by adding weight to the point they cannot lift – and then backing off just a bit and then push the maximum weight possible. This is called progressive overload and it forces the muscles to grow stronger and larger to lift the heavier weight. Working out by lifting weights at the ultimate limit of your strength is not recommended for novice weight lifters. Professionals say beginners can achieve the same results a lot safer, by progressively adding repetitions to the workout, and not lifting heavier weights. This will still fatigue muscles, wear down fibers, and result in the progressive micro trauma required to build muscle, strength and stamina.

So what does all this mean? In order for weight lifting to result in building muscle and increasing strength, you must allow the body some down time to "heal". Because it is this "healing" that is really the process of building renewed and strengthened muscle tissue. What that means is that you should not lift everyday – especially in the beginning of your weight lifting regimen. Muscle growth can take anywhere from 2 to 4 days. So beginners generally will work out every other day. The more experienced you are the longer the recovery period actually can be. Professional or very experienced weight lifters require more strength to push the limit, and causes more damage when they do, and therefore require longer time to build and repair muscles for greater strength. The pros will use a weight lifting routine that works any given specific muscle group only every 4 days.

CHAPTER 1- BASIC WEIGHTLIFTING EQUIPMENT

When it comes to exercise equipment, with the possible exception of the jump rope you really can't get much more basic than the gear you need for weight lifting. The first body builders probably just used very big rocks! But seriously, one of the nice things about weight lifting is not only is it a great way to get in shape, and build strength and self-confidence – it does not really require any real fancy or expensive equipment.

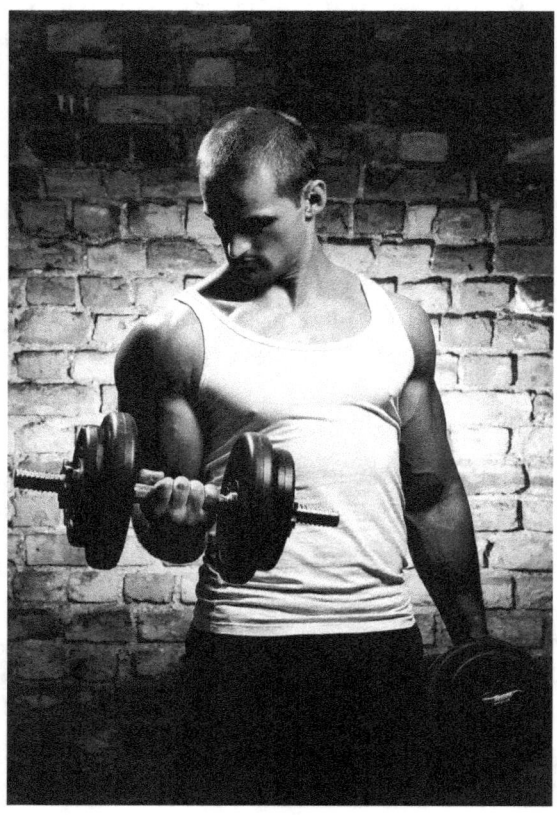

Robert Young

Now you can join a gym and have access to all the weight lifting gear you can imagine, both free weights and machines. But you can also accomplish many of the benefits of weight lifting with a basic set of barbells, dumbbells, and a good home workout regimen. Dumbbells usually are the familiar one-piece bone-shaped hand weights. Barbells are usually used for the more advanced workouts and longer muscle groups. This is the long bar with adjustable weight by adding or subtracting weighted plates. Although you can purchase a dumbbell-sized bar, and effectively use plates to make a dumbbell, generally speaking Dumbbells are fixed weights.

For basic weight lifting most pros recommend a 5-50lb Hex Dumbbell set. The hex refers to the shape of the weights – they are hexagonal rather than round, so they will not roll when you put them down. You walls and your toes will thank you. 5– 50lbHex sets can be purchased for less than 500.00 complete with racks. As far as a Barbell set goes, it depends on how much weight you want to have available to you in terms of the plates. And the nice thing about barbells is of course you can always purchase additional weight plates as you lift and increase your abilities. But a decent starter set of Barbells and plates is definitely under 200.00.

Garage sales are a great place to find barbells and plates – unfortunately people do not always stick to their commitment to lift weights. A curling bar is also a good idea. Basically a curved barbell (you can use the same plates as on your straight bar) that makes the action of doing curls easier. You also may want to pick up a weight bench. This too can often be found used. A weight bench is essential for doing many weight lifting exercises for the back and chest – and it also can be used for abdominal crunches, and triceps dips with your dumbbells.

Other accessories you may want to consider are a good pair of weight lifting gloves to protect your hands while lifting. Unless you have a back problem you already are aware of weight belts for additional support are usually not necessary for basic weight lifting workouts. In fact, some trainers so they do more harm than good because they allow a lifter to lift more than they really are physically capable of, and cause certain muscles in the forearms and lower back to receive less of a work out and less of a benefit from your weight lifting routine. Don't forget that the basic physics of weight lifting is to apply force against muscle contraction to overcome the force of gravity – that same feat can be accomplished by lifting your body weight – and if you are really on a tight budget or pressed for space a simple chin-up bar can be installed in any doorway to get in some lifting and strength training.

CHAPTER 2- HOW WEIGHTLIFTING HELPS WITH WEIGHT LOSS

Can I lose weight by lifting weights? It is a good question. And the answer is if that is the intention of your weight lifting regimen - yes. Now of course in the classic story of the "98 pound weakling" who got sand kicked in his face on the beach and then went on to become Charles Atlas – weight lifting leads to increased muscle mass and weight gain - and of course even today many people lift weights to "bulk up". But a properly designed weight lifting workout can be used to burn fat, increase metabolism and lose weight.

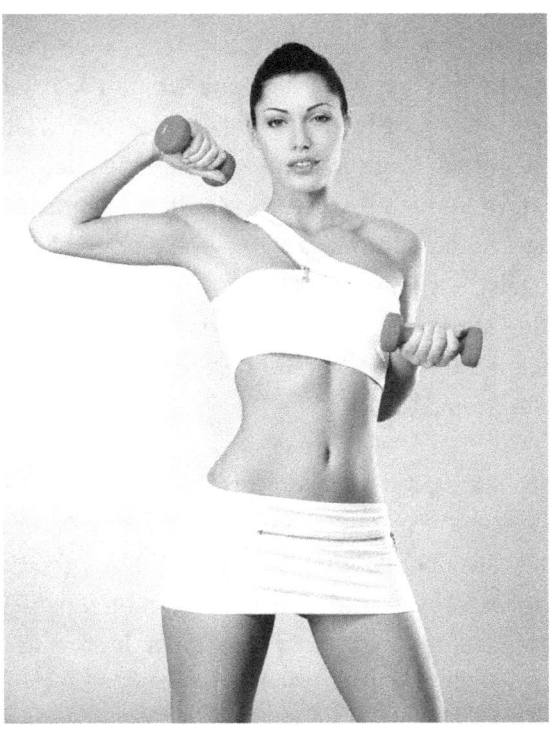

Doctors and fitness experts agree the key to effective weight loss is to rise what is called Resting Metabolism. Resting Metabolism Rate (RMR) is the rate at which your body consumes fuel when at rest. That fuel is better known as calories. Do you know where the bulk of calories is burnt or used in the body? It'he lean muscle mass. Muscle is active tissue, muscles even at rest burn calories – fat does not. The more lean muscle mass you have, the more calories you burn. What is the best way to build lean muscle mass – lifting weights of course!

This is why diet alone, never leads to permanent weight loss; diet without exercise does nothing to increase RMR. And even the exercises usually associated with slimming down, like aerobics and other cardio workouts; also do little to raise RMR – that is why fitness gurus all suggest adding weight lifting to any exercise program designed for effective and permanent weight loss. This is true for men as well as women. Many women fear weight lifting because they are afraid they will get "too bulky" or "too manly". This is simply not so, Mother Nature has seen to that. Most women just do not have enough testosterone (which speeds and enhances muscle growth, actually making it easier for men to raise their RMR, sorry gals) – to develop a "manly physique". Remember, we are not talking about a heavy 2 hour a day pumping iron session. As part of a regimen to raise RMR, moderate weight lifting 2 – 3 times a week is all it should take.

Start out with a weight that is comfortable for you and that you can lift in any given exercise 8-12 times or repetitions. If the muscles do not become noticeably fatigued by the 12th time, the weight is too light, gradually increase until the first signs of fatigue come in at around that 12th rep. To build the most lean mass, gradually increase the weight by about 10% each time you can do the 12 reps. Remember, weight lifting is designed to raise RMR and build lean muscle mass as an adjunct to cardio, not as a replacement.

Robert Young

They work arm and arm, cardio to burn fat – weight lifting to build muscle mass and increase RMR.

The bottom line is dieting slows metabolism – weight lifting increases it. Dieting, plus weight lifting leads to a slimmer healthier you.

CHAPTER 3- PROPER WEIGHTLIFTING TECHNIQUES

How to Squat

To achieve the proper benefit for any given weight lift exercise you must know the proper techniques and do it right. Incorrect lifting technique can work the wrong muscle groups, or worse result in strain or other injuries. The idea of "no pain – no gain" refers to the burn or the tingle you get when you have worked a muscle to the point that will result in its coming back stronger. Weight lifting is not supposed to hurt, and if it does you are either using inappropriate amount of weight or improper technique.

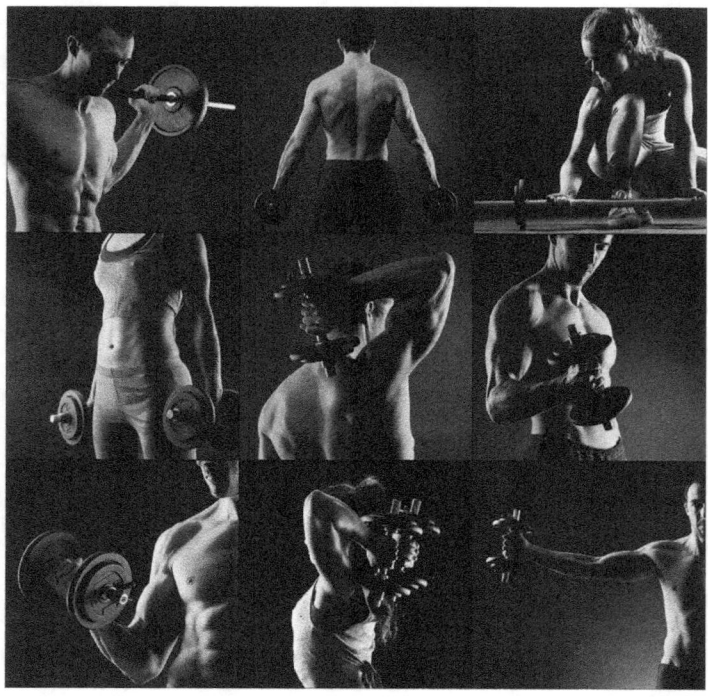

Robert Young

One of the most common weight lifting repetition exercises is the Squat. The Squat, which can be done with Free Weights or Machines, is one of the best weight lifting exercises there is to build lower body and leg strength. The squat is a weight lifting exercise primarily targeting the quadriceps (thigh muscles) and the gluts (rear end). But when done correctly, it also works out the hamstrings, the calves, and the lower back. Weight lifters have called the Squat "The King of All Exercises" because it works so many muscles at one time and so quickly builds muscle mass. Ironman Tri-Athlete, Ray Fautex says that if you only had 15 minutes a day to do one exercise make it squats.

The squat is done by bending at the knees and hips and lowering the torso between the legs, and then returning to a standing position. The torso should remain as upright as possible during the bend. When doing squats, keep your back straight. Your feet should be about shoulder length apart. Keep your toes pointed forward. Try it a few times with no weight.

If it feels difficult you are probably doing it right. It is absolutely critical to keep the back straight during squats or serious injury to the lower back can occur. If you already have a weakened lower back due to injury, a weight belt could be worn during squats to help support the lower back. Feet should remain flat on the floor. To maintain proper balance during the upward motion of the squat, force should be exerted from the heel of the foot and not the toes. If squatting with a particularly heavy weight you should use a squat cage, or have a spotter to help you return the barbell to a safe resting position after the squats.

The most common squat is the back squat – were the barbell is held behind the head, across the upper back. But there are dozens of variants such as the Hack Squat where the weight is held behind the legs. The Overhead Squat, which is my particular favorite –

squatting while holding the barbell at full extension over your head. There are several Squats where you hold the barbell in front of you like the aptly named Front Squat, where it is gripped with your arms folded across your chest, or the Zercher Squat, where it is held in the crook of the arms.

Squatting is a great weight lifting exercise, but by its very nature a very rigorous one. It is recommended that a squat be learned from an experienced weight lifter or professional trainer to avoid potential serious injury.

The Deadlift

In weight lifting it is important to know the proper techniques to achieve the desired benefit of a given weight lift exercise. Lifting incorrectly not only can work the wrong muscles, but also may cause muscle strain or other injuries. Despite the popular motivational expression "no pain – no gain," weight lifting when done correctly should not hurt, if you are experiencing physical pain during or after a weight lifting workout, chances are you are using the wrong amount of weight or incorrect technique.

The Deadlift is a popular weight lifting exercise in competition and for professional and personal training. It is the classic weightlifting technique where one grasps a barbell that is on the floor from a squatting position and stands up bringing the barbell to just past the knees. It is the ultimate "test of strength" and is the key movement in competitive Powerlifting. While you start from a "squatted" position A Deadlift is unlike a Squat or most other weight lifting techniques for that matter, because as its name implies you are lifting a "dead weight". In other words a weight that is not already in motion or otherwise already off the ground.

It is for this reason that it really puts the muscles to the test, and can also be quite risky if done wrong. The Deadlift works just about every muscle group of the lower body, including the abs, the lower back and the back. Other muscle groups involved include the hips, thighs, hamstrings, calves and glutes. To some degree the Deadlift also works the trapeziums (upper back and holders) and the forearms.

To Deadlift, grab the bar with a comfortable grip; the legs should be shoulder length apart; lower body into a squatting position with hips parallel to the floor with the back straight and the eyes looking forward. Tighten your stomach muscles, and raise yourself and the bar "pushing" with your leg muscles and extending your hips, you are not lifting the weight with your arms or your back. The bar should come to a position above your knees and in front of the hips.

Do not round your shoulders. Return the bar slowly to the ground and repeat. The biggest mistake people make in a Deadlift that can cause serious injury is trying to lift with the arms, back, or other muscles of the upper body. While some of these groups will be working in a Deadlift, the Deadlift is not an upper body weightlifting exercise. To avoid this it is helpful for the lifter to envision trying to push your legs and hips through the floor rather than pulling up on the bar with your arms and back.

The serious risk of improper lifting in a dead lift is back injury. It is imperative to keep the back straight during a dead lift. If you do not this can put stress on the disks and lead to all manner of back problems. A lifting belt could stabilize the lower back and is a good idea if you already have a back condition; however, some pros say that lifting belts prevent you from strengthening the very areas that are in need of help from people with back pain.

There are a few variations in weight lifting of the Deadlift, such as the Romanian Deadlift, which is not really a Deadlift at all since in this variation after initial lift, you do not return the bar to the floor. It is designed to work more of the thighs and hamstrings.

The world record for the Deadlift is held by weight lifter Andrew Bolton of Great Britain who pulled 1003 pounds, the first ever Deadlift over 1000 pounds.

CHAPTER 4- OVERALL FITNESS AND WEIGHTLIFTING

Weight lifting is probably the single most effective exercise you can do to improve health and general fitness. Weight lifting raises your metabolism. Weightlifting builds strength and self-confidence. Weight lifting can improve your game no matter what sport you are active in. Weight lifting improves cardio function and heart health. Weight lifting can even strengthen bones and lessen or prevent the symptoms associated with osteoporosis.

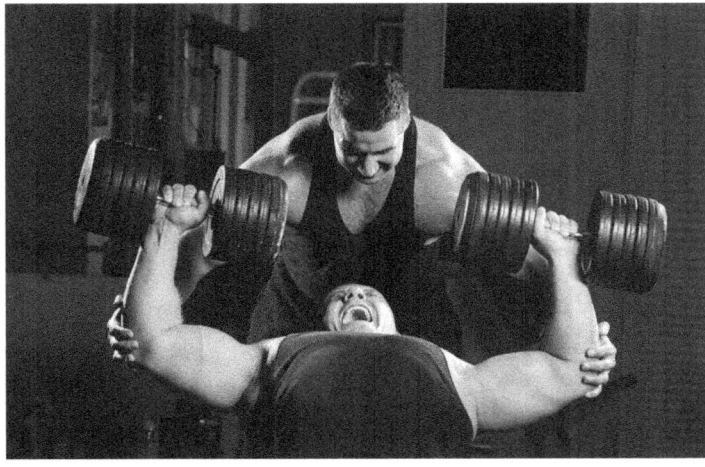

Big or small, short or tall, anyone can benefit and benefit greatly from weight lifting. As we age our metabolism slows down and we lose lean muscle mass and bone density. Loss of lean muscle mass leads to even slower metabolism, and this becomes a vicious cycle leading to an overweight and sedentary lifestyle which brings with it a whole host of other health problems. Now I am not saying that lifting weights and weight training can reverse the ageing process, but it can break this cycle, and make you feel fit and keep you fit at any age. Just ask Jack LaLanne, still going "strong" and he is over 90 years old.

One of the hardest parts of any exercise program is motivation to keep going. It is easier to stay motivated with weightlifting and weight training than most other exercise because you can see and feel the result in just a short time. Weight lift for only a few weeks and you will start to see an immediate increase in your strength and stamina by 20 to 40%. And this will not only be in the gym, suddenly all those grocery bags you carry home from the store or your kids are going to feel much lighter. Increased strength and power will improve any sport you are into. Stronger leg muscles will allow you to run faster. Stronger upper body and can hit a ball harder or throw further. Weightlifting and strength training improve stamina overall, and stronger muscles and bones can take more of a pounding so lifting weights can help prevent other sports related injuries.

Of course weight training will help you look better. And many people start lifting only to improve their physique and physical appearance. They do not even realize all of the other benefits one gets from sculpting a toned and defined body by weight lifting. While some fitness experts argue that Aerobic exercise is better to improve cardiovascular health than weight training, studies have proven that cardiac output increases during weight lifting. And of course it is a physiological fact that the heart and lungs support all muscle function, so when the muscles are taxed during weightlifting their support system is also getting a workout. That is why today most fitness experts suggest that you engage in an exercise program that includes at least some weight lifting combined with cardio, even a few days a week, for total overall good health and fitness.

CHAPTER 5- BODY MASS INDEX- A CLOSER LOOK

One of the ways that medical professionals determine if you are overweight is by a rating called body mass index. BMI is an approximate measure of body fat based on weight and height proportion. BMI was designed to get an approximation or snapshot of body fat – it can overestimate Body fat in those with a lot of lean muscle mass, like weightlifters. BMI is calculated by taking your weight in pounds, multiplying by 703 and dividing that number by your height in inches squared. Compare the results as follows:

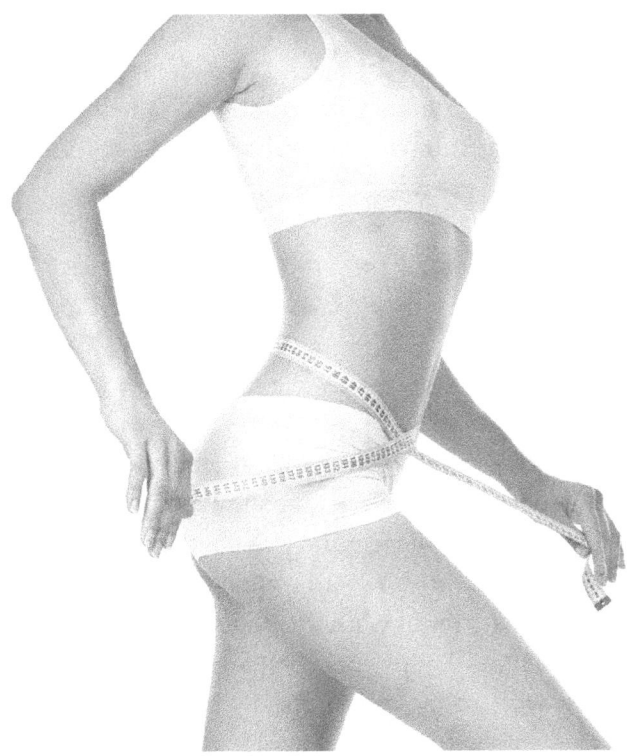

BMI   WEIGHT STATUS

Below 18.5   Underweight

18.5 -24.9   Normal

25 - 29.9   Overweight

30 & Above   Obese

Now, while it is true that professional weightlifters and especially professional bodybuilders whose regimen and diet is specifically programmed to increase lean muscle for "show" and eliminate as much body fat as possible – can have an inaccurate reading on their BMI. A competitive bodybuilder, for example, has on average only 4% body fat! But for most of us, if you have not already picked up the sport of weight lifting – and you hit in the 25 or over range on that chart, the truth is there is no better way to lower that BMI and get in shape the weight lifting.

Weightlifting eliminates most of the problems of yo-yo dieting by building lean muscle mass and increasing metabolism. Especially for ageing baby boomers that see those BMI numbers creeping up and want to do something about it – weight lifting is the way to go.

For weight control, it is best to combine weight lifting with cardiovascular workouts, and of course healthy eating. Foods rich in fiber and whole grains and low in fat are the keys to effective weight loss when combined with weight training and exercise. And don't forget to also drink a lot of water. It is important if you really want to lower your BMI and get in better shape that you combine your weight lifting with cardio workouts. In the first place you should never lift weights without doing some kind of cardio warm up first – just to get the heart and lungs pumping. Also, if you are really weightlifting to sculpt a defined and toned body – you need the cardio to burn calories and fat.

In developing a weight lifting routine designed to maximize health, strength, build muscle and reduce your BMI – it is important not to over train. That means rotate your muscle groups. And you also need to be aware of primary and secondary muscle groups. What that means is that there are weightlifting exercises that are designed to work a primary muscle group, but since almost all muscles are interconnected, they also will train a secondary muscle group.

This is the very reason why weightlifting gives you so much "bang for the buck" and a total body workout. For example, just about every lift to build chest and shoulders also works the triceps. So if you do triceps on one day, followed by chest the next, and the shoulders the following you will overwork and over train the triceps. A good rotation is or split would be:

Monday - Chest/Triceps

Tuesday – Break

Wednesday – Back/Biceps

Thursday – Break

Friday – Legs/Shoulders

Saturday & Sunday Break

Strength Training Tips

In many places you will hear or see weightlifting and strength training used as if they are the same thing. They technically are not. Weightlifting is a type of strength training, but it is not the only one. The whole idea of strength training is to build muscle mass. Muscle mass is built by forcing muscles to work harder against an opposing force. In weightlifting that force is gravity. You use your muscles to lift either a free weight or weights on a machine to overcome gravity. But there are other types of strength training too – such as resistance strength training, in which you use the muscle to overcome resistance like that of a resistance band, or resistance machine that uses a series of pulleys. Or Isometric strength training that pits one muscle against another.

Still most fitness professionals agree one of the best methods of building muscle is to strength train through weightlifting. And for the purposes of most discussions about how we build muscle and the many benefits thereof, strength training and weight lifting can be considered interchangeable. In fact prior to modern times where much more has been learned about physiology and exercise, and other methods of strength training exercises have been developed, strength training and weight training were pretty much interchangeable terminologies.

Regardless of what you call it strength training and/or weightlifting provides significant health benefits. Strength training builds muscle, strengthens bones and ligaments, and adds to overall fitness and well-being. The key to using weightlifting to increase strength is to use the concept of progressive resistance. You need to continue to tax the muscles by increasing the force they need to work against overtime to continue to build up and gain strength. In weightlifting this is accomplished by either adding more weight or increasing repetitions. Weightlifting is also a great way to strength train because weight lifting exercises, either with free weights or machines have been designed to work targeted and specific muscle groups. So if you want to add strength to your legs because you are a soccer player, you can target leg-lifting exercises, and still receive many secondary benefits of weightlifting and general strength training.

Weightlifting is not however the same thing as Bodybuilding. Popularized by the Movie "Pumping Iron" and rise in fame of Arnold Schwarzenegger, bodybuilding uses similar techniques to weight lifting and carries many of the same benefits, but it is sport with different goals. Most bodybuilders train for open competition, so their goal is to maximize muscularity and minimize body fat. Competitive body builders have from 2- 4% total body fat. A weight lifter or weight trainer on the other hand, is primarily concerned with increasing strength and stamina, and is not too concerned with reducing body fat to below normal levels, and will wind up looking and feeling good by doing that.

CHAPTER 6- HOW WEIGHTLIFTING AFFECTS OVERALL HEALTH

Whether your 8 or 80 years of age, weightlifting can be used to improve your overall health. While at one time it was thought that children should avoid lifting weight as exercise because it can cause damage to their maturing bones, and that seniors are just too weak and frail to weight lift. Both of these ideas have proven unfounded. Weightlifting when done correctly can help anyone get and keep fit. There has been very little evidence of bone growth plate damage in children who weight train properly, and seniors well into their 80's and 90's have shown to actually reduce some of the bone loss that comes with aging by working out with weights.

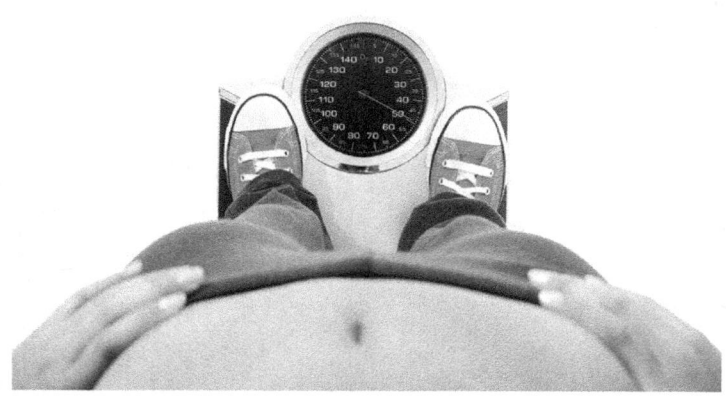

Weight lifting has a multitude of benefits that do not start and end with the obvious of increased strength and more lean muscle mass. We know that increased muscle mass increases your metabolism. Increased metabolism helps you lose weight and keep it off. Weight lifting is also a great natural anti-depressant. It relieves stress like any strong work out by raising the level of endorphins like dopamine and serotonin, which are known to fight feelings of depression and anxiety.

Basic weight lifting techniques and workouts are usually what are called isotonic exercises, because the muscles are used to apply force to push or pull a weighted object. That object could be anything, but most commonly we are talking about barbells or dumbbells, or weight machines. Weight lifting exercises to gain strength and improve health can be isolation exercises or compound exercises. An isolation exercise is one that is designed to work out or build a specific muscle or muscle group, like a leg lift. Compound exercises are those weigh lifts that are designed to work several muscle groups. Inclined leg presses, where you use both legs to press out to move a weight while reclining on a weight bench is a compound exercise because it involves the quads, the hips, hamstrings, and glutes and even can strengthen the knee joints. That is one of the greatest health benefits of weight lifting – many single exercises can be used to work groups of muscles, and produce a great total body workout. Compound exercises are the best to develop increased strength for overall health and daily activities. The muscles worked out in most compound weight lifting exercises most closely resemble the pushing, pulling, bending and lifting we do in our everyday activities, and will make these tasks much easier after just a few weeks of weightlifting.

Most of the common weight lifting exercises you are familiar with like the Squat, Deadlift, and Bench Press are compound exercises. Another example of an Isolation Exercise would be the Curl for Biceps. Isolation exercises can be helpful if you want to target a specific muscle group and improve performance for a given sport like your golf or tennis swing, or improving your forearms to help carry around your four year old, as my wife recently discovered!

Heart Health

Conventional wisdom has been that the best exercise to improve heart health and maintain a healthy cardiovascular system and thereby reducing the risk of stroke and heart attack were aerobic or so called cardio workouts. Weight lifting has traditionally been considered an anaerobic exercise, and as such was not thought to be the best choice for heart health. However that is no longer the thinking. Many medical professionals and personal trainers recognize the benefits weightlifting has on the heart and lungs, especially when combined with more traditional cardio workouts.

Up until recently cardiologists actually discouraged their patients from weight training and weightlifting that view is changing. The American Heart Association published recent evidence that shows the benefits to the heart of working out with weights. The reversal of opinion is not only because physiologists now recognize that there is indeed an aerobic component to weightlifting exercises, but because of the overall improvement in condition and body changes that weightlifting and building muscle create. It has been found that increasing muscle mass and strength actually lowers Resting Metabolism, and resting blood pressure.

While the benefits of building muscle to the body's most important muscle, the heart – are becoming readily apparent for any healthy person – for the heart patient weightlifting and resistance training can be very important to preventing future heart attacks or other cardiac episodes. It is all about being in better condition and being stronger. It's not brain surgery but it is basic heart science. If you have a weak heart even simple tasks like walking up stairs lifting groceries, even walking can put a strain on it.

If you are stronger from building lean muscle mass these tasks become that much simpler, your heart doesn't have to work so hard. Studies have also shown that when people lifting weight were monitored for cardiac output the heart pumped stronger and faster. Like any muscle this builds stronger walls in the ventricle, the pumping part of the heart. Strong ventricles mean the heart can pump more efficiently, and effectively lowers resting heart rate, which can lower blood pressure, one of the main contributing factors to heart attack and stroke.

Of course gaining a healthy heart is not the only benefit of weightlifting. Most people who have heart problems are also overweight or struggling with some of the other problems of obesity like diabetes. Weightlifting is a great way to lose weight and keep it off by raising your metabolism and making your body burn calories more efficiently. While minute for minute anaerobic exercises like weightlifting will not burn as much as an aerobic exercise like biking or jogging, in other words15 minute on a stationary bike initially burn far more calories than 15 minutes of weightlifting. However it's been found that up to two hours after a 15 minute weightlifting workout, the body continues to burn calories as the muscles remain in an agitated state. The American Heart Association now recommends a 30 minute aerobic workout 6 times a week, and adding a weightlifting session of at least 15 minutes 3 times a week.

Joint Health

With our ageing baby boomer population, joint pain and joint problems such as arthritis are rapidly becoming major health concerns. Knee, hip and other "load bearing" joint surgeries are becoming increasingly more common. But did you know that a regimen of exercise that includes weightlifting and nutritional supplements like Glucosamine has actually helped some people avoid surgery?

Strength Training for Beginners

First up we must dispel the myth that working-out with weights can cause joint pain. Now I am not saying that no one has ever left a gym with a sore knee, or shoulder, or elbow, quite the contrary people often do. But if that is caused by your weightlifting routine you are probably doing something wrong. Chances are you are not warming up properly prior to weightlifting, lifting with poor technique, or too much weight, or are not allowing enough time for your joints to recuperate after sets. Here we are discussing the joint pain that can and does occur from every day "wear and tear", Osteoarthritis or other conditions. Proper weight training has been found to actually improve joint health, return functionality and decrease this pain.

A recent study released in the October 2006 issue of Arthritis Care and Research followed two groups of patients with knee arthritis. One group was given a regular series of Range of Motion Exercises the other a regular routine of Strength Training Exercises, that included weightlifting routines to strengthen the quadriceps and other leg muscles. All patients in the weightlifting group reported less pain then in the ROM group, and more importantly X-rays of those in the Strength Training Group verified that the progression of their arthritis had slowed.

Regular exercise of the joints replenishes joint lubricants and builds cartilage. Weightlifting increases the muscles around joints. Stronger muscles from weightlifting exercises offer more support to the joints. From the process of weightlifting you become physically stronger. This means you can participate in more activities, which make your joints healthier. We already know how weight training builds muscle and how that can improve your overall health and help you lose weight. All orthopedic specialists agree a sure way to reduce joint pain and improve joint health is to lose weight, and ease some of the burden on those weight-bearing joints like the hip or knees.

Simple common weight training exercises have been found to be the best to reduce joint pain of the hips and lower extremities, such as Squats and Leg Extensions. If you are not already weightlifting just as a matter of course to improve health, and are experiencing knee or hip pain, now is a great time to start. Many Americans have totally eliminated their need for ant-inflammatory drugs and other medications to manage their joint pain through weightlifting and strength training. And once you have eliminated your joint pain and start to realize all the other benefits from working out with weights, you can be well on your way on the road to better health and better fitness all around.

Back Injuries

Weightlifting is a great way to get in shape and stay in shape. However like many physical activities it is not without its set of risks. Probably the most common injury from weightlifting is back injury. But while back injuries are a potential risk from weightlifting, if they do occur most often they are from poor technique or other errors made by the lifter that can be easily avoided.

There are several possible back injuries that can occur during weightlifting, the most common are stress fractures that occur when flexing the muscles, tendons and ligaments of the back against resistance such as one does during weightlifting. These types of injuries are most commonly caused by improper technique during squats, deadlifts and clean and jerks. Older people who may already be suffering from degenerative disc disease or people who may already be recuperating from a back injury are particularly susceptible to weightlifting related back injuries. There are several ways to avoid back injuries while weightlifting:

- Know your limitations, do not lift beyond your weight max based on your body condition
- For many exercises it is easier and for those with an injured or weakened back especially, safer to work out using weight machines over free weights
- If you do choose to use free weights, make sure you work with a spotter
- While the use of weight belts for most lifters generally is agreed to have little value, for those with an injured back they can be useful in preventing further injury. Check with your doctor or personal trainer if they think you should use a black belt.
- Do not attempt to do the weightlifting exercises that most often result in back injury i.e.: squats, deadlifts, and clean and jerks, without proper training and or supervision.

We've spoken a lot about preventing back injuries while weightlifting, what about returning to lifting after a back injury, one that may or may not have even been caused by lifting? First off you can and will return, but do not expect to return exactly where you left off. You may be able to ease back into you exact routine; you may have to modify your routine to suit your current condition.

Only your trainer or spine care professional will be able to accurately advise you. Most fitness pros agree however that after an injury re-establishing that "mind muscle link" that gets the body back into muscle building mode is critically important, and the hardest aspect to the road back. It is best to start slow and ease your body back into bodybuilding gear when coming back from an injury, just as you would do from taking any significant break in your regular weightlifting routine.

CHAPTER 7- SHOULD KIDS LIFT WEIGHTS

There was a time when it was debatable whether kids should lift weights and strength train. The controversy stemmed from the fact that the epiphyseal plates or so-called growth plates, that allow a child to grow, are not closed completely in children and youths. The open distance in these plates is what allows for growth and the thinking was that weightlifting, and certain other forms of physical activity can close these structures prematurely, and impact a child's growth and development. Recent studies have shown that there is no clinical evidence of weightlifting in children causing growth plate injuries. And in fact most personal trainers and family physicians agree that weightlifting and strength training is beneficial to children.

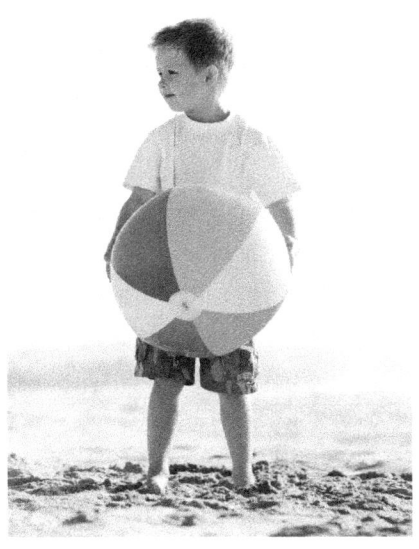

Obesity, especially obesity in children is rampant in this country. Weightlifting fats fight. We know that. Building lean muscle mass is the best way for children or anybody to get rid of fat. Weight training and weightlifting provides a routine and discipline that many children crave and need. Weightlifting in children builds not only muscle but also self-esteem. It teaches children at an early age respect for their bodies and sets in motion good nutrition and good health habits for a lifetime. Speaking from personal experience, this former proverbial "98 pound weakling" who was the target of many a school yard bullies never had his lunch money stolen again after I began weightlifting and strength training in the 5th grade, at the advice of my grandfather, a former Golden Glove Boxer.

The American Society of Pediatrics recently issued guidelines for strength training and weightlifting in adolescents. The report concluded that weightlifting indeed presents no harm to adolescents (other than the same general risks of injury to any weightlifter) and in fact it does lead to increased strength and muscle growth in adolescents and pre-adolescents. The guidelines went on to say that teens and preteens should not lift to their maximum to avoid potential injury to growth plates, and that they should lift a weight that they could comfortably do 12 –15 repetitions with on a given weightlifting exercise.

Now no one is suggesting that your child especially a young one start training like a power lifter. However, studies have shown that children as young as 8 doing a little strength training about 100 minutes a week, not at the maximum weight, but at that 10-12 rep range, saw a drastic increase in strength. It was reported that children in the study, which monitored 8-12 year olds, also showed improvements in eating habits. And interestingly enough parents in the study also reported a noticeable improvement in the behavior and attitude of their children.

CHAPTER 8- WEIGHT LIFTING FOR THE WOMAN

For many years it was believed that weightlifting was only an activity to be done by men. And even then only by a special breed of males, who wanted to become superhuman examples of human perfection. Even as over the past few decades it has come to be generally accepted that weightlifting is something that has benefits for men other than the muscle beach crowd, still it has generally been looked upon as a male activity. Women fear weightlifting.

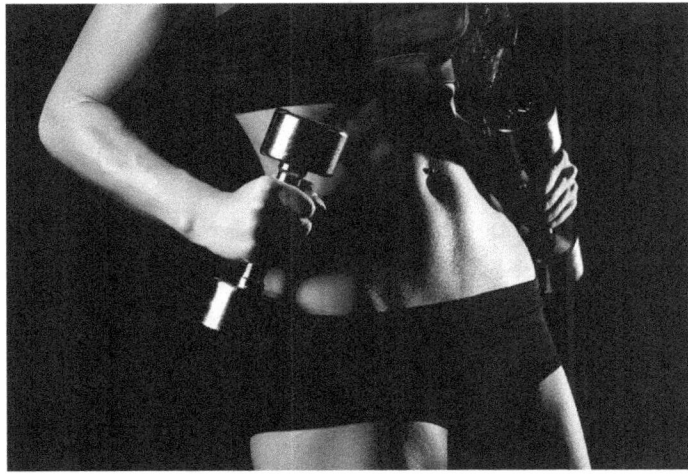

They think it will make them look too big, or "like men" They think weightlifting is only for the most athletic of women. Not true. Indeed there is a sport of female bodybuilding – but these women will be the first to tell you that they need to work extremely hard, probably twice or three times as hard, to gain that kind of physique as their male counter parts. Why? A simple biological fact – women do not make enough testosterone to build muscle as big or as quickly as men do.

So don't worry about it ladies you can work out with weights and get phenomenal health benefits like losing weight and looking younger – yes I said "losing weight" and "looking younger" – by weightlifting! Lean muscle burns calories. Lean muscle is sexy. There is absolutely no reason why fitness conscious women today mostly restrict their workouts to just cardio and aerobics. Women can benefit from lean muscle mass as much as men.

Biological fact number two – we lose muscle mass as we age, do nothing to replace it; we lose strength and tone and look and feel older. Most Women also know that they are more susceptible to bone density loss than men, so they take calcium supplements. Weightlifting strengthens and builds not only muscle but bones. Studies in women have shown that resistance training such as weightlifting cannot only prevent but in some cases can reverse the effects of osteoporosis.

Ladies you want shape – you want a figure – building up the muscles of your shoulders and back will make your waist look smaller. And let's not forget about what weightlifting can do for the old Gluteus Maximus. You really want "Buns of Steel"? – Pump Iron!

Trainers do not suggest that women give up aerobics altogether. In fact a workout regimen that combines traditional cardio-aerobics and weightlifting is ideal. However one more point to note a recent study following women age 24-34 conducted by the Jon Hopkins University found that women who lifted weights continued to burn calories sometimes up to 2 hours longer after the exercise then women who did a comparable period of aerobics.

CHAPTER 9- HOW TO USE WEIGHTLIFTING TO BULK UP

When people think of weightlifting and building muscle they usually are thinking of two things, "Bulk" and "definition". People will throw around words like I am interested in "building muscle" or and this is especially true of woman, say I don't want to get bulky I just want "to get toned". Further they think bodybuilding is going for "definition and or tone" and weightlifting for "Muscle or Bulk". Well a lot of these terms get misused, even in professional lifting and body building magazines. The truth is that weightlifting, any kind of weight lifting will do both - grow your muscles and tone you muscles. When they talk about definition, or what most people refer to as "Muscle Tone" they really are talking about the muscles you can see, like the six pack abs or bulging pecks. Well in that case Body builders are the ones that are most concerned with showing off their physique as they weightlift for a visual competition – and they know that the way to get "sculpted" and show those muscles has much less to do with how you weightlift as it is with reducing body fat percentage, no muscles, no matter how "toned" will show under a layer of fat.

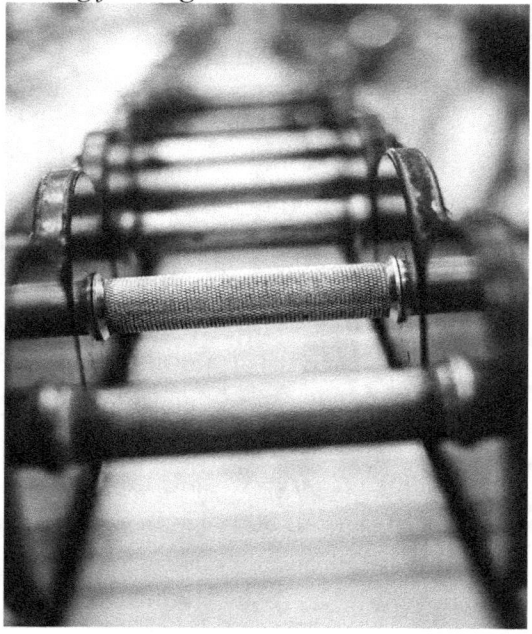

But if you want to "get big" or weightlift for quote/unquote bulk here is the safe and effective way to do it. It's all about being able to constantly push your muscles to the point that they will continue to grow to their maximum potential which ultimately is determined by your genes. It involves a couple of basic principles, details will vary as you tailor a program to your specific goals and body type, but so long as you train smart, eat right, and get the right amount rest to renew and rebuild – you will bulk up. Period! It's that simple.

First let's set a baseline. Get a tape measure and measure you biceps, quads, abs, and every area you want to "bulk up". Also take a picture of yourself. You know all those classic before and after pictures? Follow a program of sensible weightlifting keeping those three basic principles in mind: lift smart, eat right, rest – and you will be that "after guy" (or gal). Set realistic goals for strength or muscle growth. If you can add from a half a pound to a pound of lean muscle mass every week that is good.

A good routine for bulking up means that you should not work any given muscle group more than once a week. The key is to let the body heal and repair that is how muscle growth occurs. When you start lifting of course you will feel sore for the next day or two. Some suggest that you should go back to work that group soon as the pain is gone, but there has been a lot of fitness and medical pros that have said that healing and repairing of muscle tissue that leads to growth and increased strength doesn't happen until after the pain has subsided.

The right diet for "bulking up" when lifting should have a ratio of 40% Protein, 40% Carbs, and 20% Fat. Stick with complex carbs, avoid sugars and processes carbs, and stick with whole grains. As far as Fats go you know the drill, avoid the bad fats, hydrogenated oils, and Trans fats – and stick with good fats like those found in nuts.

Building Definition

"Definition" ironically is one of the most improperly defined words in weightlifting and fitness. It is the most misunderstood and misused term out there. I have even seen professional fitness and weightlifting magazines throw around the terms "Tone" and "Definition" indiscriminately and more often than not incorrectly.

When most people use the term "tone" or "definition" they are using it in opposition to the term "bulk". They think bodybuilders are "bulky" the body of a gymnast "toned" and "defined." Poppycock! Nothing can be further from the truth. In fact it is the body builder whose ultimate goal is true "definition". Definition in its purest sense is being able to see clearly "defined" and separated muscle groups. This is exactly what a bodybuilder strives for and competes with.

Yet people think weightlifting especially heavy weightlifting is not for "definition". You will constantly hear people in gyms saying they are not lifting heavy because they are only looking to "tone up" not "get big". Women especially will not weightlift or only lift with repetition after repetition of light weights because they think this will give them "tone and definition". Definition by its true "definition" is less about what weightlifting routines you do, and what weight you work out with, then what you do about reducing your body fat percentage. Muscle cannot be "defined" or look "toned" — if it is hiding under body fat. This is why bodybuilders go for percentage of total body fat in the 2-4% range. And getting to that kind of "definition" is more a function of diet, than any specific kind of weightlifting.

So what are the best weightlifting routines to "tone" "sculpt" or "define" your muscles? All of them! Weightlifting does one thing and one thing only; by pushing muscles to the point of stress it makes the muscle react to the stress by growing bigger and stronger. And yes bigger and stronger means tighter and firmer, but if you want to see that, or want the person sitting down the bar from you to see that, you must reduce the fat. Any weightlifting routine has a fat burning component, and muscle in and of itself burns fat, but if you want to get rid of the fat and be more "defined" that will come from cardio — bike riding, jogging, swimming etc., it's that simple. You want to feel and look your best, want to be strong and look great in spandex? Then weightlift to build lean muscle and eat right and do cardio and aerobics to reduce fat.

CHAPTER 10- DOES GENETICS PLAY A ROLE IN HOW YOU BUILD MUSCLE?

Nature or Nurture- It has been a debate that comes into play in just about every aspect of human behavior or ability. How strong, how smart, how fast we are, or can be -are we a product of our environment or genes? --Or both? Weightlifters, body builders and fitness pros, are no strangers to this debate.

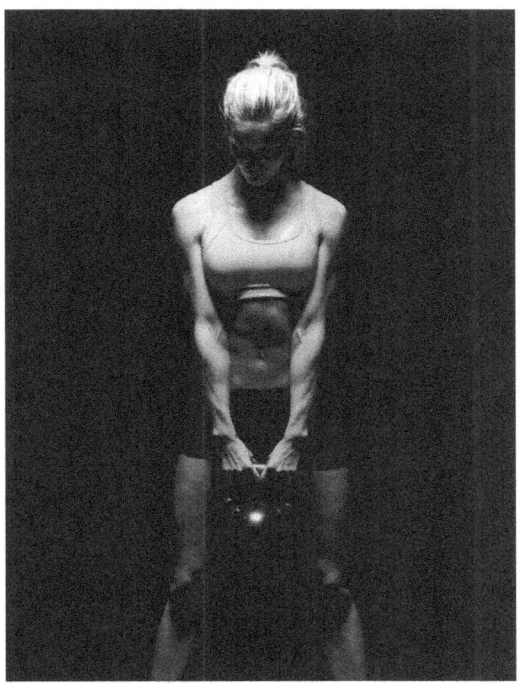

Anyone can build muscle and reduce fat by lifting weights. So if the question is will your genes determine if you will get stronger or bigger by weightlifting – the answer is no. It does not matter what your genetic proclivities are you will improve you physique and your health by weightlifting. Ultimately how big, or how strong you will get is determined by genetics. This is why you can take any two people, with the possible exception of identical twins, put them side by side in the gym, give them exactly the same routines for the same amount of weeks – and they will undoubtedly build muscle and burn fat at different rates.

We all know that person, whether they are weight lifters or not - that just seems to be able to eat whatever they want, and stay lean and muscular, never seem to put on weight. While there are others, probably most of us actually, that "just look at food" and you put on fat. This is truly a genetic factor. There are people known as mesomorphs that just have a genetic predisposition towards high metabolic rates – they burn fat easily and build lean muscle easily – so yes such people could be considered "natural bodybuilders".

So what does this mean as far as weight training goes? Not much really. If you are getting into weightlifting for good health, increased strength and stamina – it doesn't matter if you are a man, a woman, 8 or eighty. No matter what your genetic make-up is you will benefit from weightlifting and building muscle mass to your maximum potential given your genes and your lifestyle. If on the other hand you dream of being a professional bodybuilder or weightlifter then you must consider more closely the hand your genes may have dealt you. Someone who is 5.1 could be very athletic and could become very good at basketball – but it is very unlikely he will ever be able to play starting Center for the Lakers. It is just as unlikely a person with a smaller genetic frame can become a champion bodybuilder. The nature of bodybuilding competitions and what judges usually look for give a major advantage to bigger taller men and women. And the aforementioned "mesomorphic" types will have a much easier time in training and getting down to the 2-3% body fat champion bodybuilders want to be at.

Robert Young

Bottom line; don't give much thought as to what lies in your genetic makeup. Train hard; push yourself to your limits every day. Follow a good regimen of weightlifting at least 3- 4 days a week, eat right, get plenty of rest, do cardio as well. Look in the mirror in a year or two – and I'm sure you will be very pleased at who is starring back. Certainly you will probably feel better and look better in your "jeans" then most people around you - no matter what's in their "genes".

CHAPTER 11- WEIGHTLIFTING AND CROSS TRAINING

Weightlifting in and of itself is a great sport. But no matter what sport you are into, or whatever you may be training for, there is not a game on the planet that weightlifting cannot improve. We all know how weightlifting can improve general health and fitness, the body benefits in so many ways be increasing strength and muscle mass. But because of the very nature of weightlifting, and the ability to target specific muscle groups with specific exercises, you can cross train by weightlifting to strengthen arms, legs or any other part of the body to perk up your game.

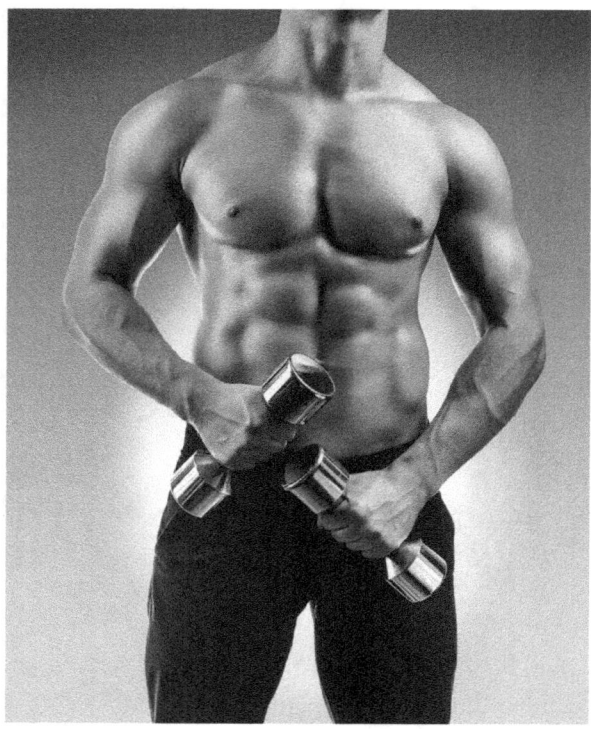

All pro athletes will weight lift as some part of their training routine. Obviously power hitters and other baseball players improve upper body strength with weight training. Ironman triathletes workout with weights doing squats and deadlifts to enhance lower body and leg strength to help in swimming and biking, and not to mention to improve stamina. Track and field stars will weight lift and weight train because of the way weightlifting promotes lean muscle mass and low body fat percentage. Winter sports are no exception, speed skaters and skiers alike know the benefits of leg lifts and leg presses. And of course football players and wrestlers will strength train and use weightlifting routines and techniques that are almost indistinguishable from a bodybuilders or power lifters.

So whether you are a pro, semi-pro or someone just trying to get in shape, however you train or workout you are not getting the max if you are not weightlifting too. Cross training just makes sense on so many levels. Variety is the spice of life and so it is true for working out. You will improve health, strength and stamina by cross training No one exercise even weightlifting can "do it all". While of course I have a certain bias toward weightlifting and feel it is the number one all- purpose way to live a happy and healthy life, even lifters have to "cross train". Just for healthy and safe lifting you know we all recommend doing 15 – 20 minutes of aerobic exercise prior to ever lift session. That right there is "cross training". Also if you really want to get and keep a lean and mean physique, weightlifting alone won't do it. It doesn't matter how tight you make that six pack – no one will see how ripped it is if it hiding under a layer of body fat. Cross training with cardio will help to burn fat.

Now I know a lot of you get really psyched up about lifting, and there is no greater natural high then after you get those endorphins flowing after a good pumping session, but let's face it, weightlifting, like any exercise routine, if you do the same thing over and over again can get a little boring. Cross training gives you the opportunity to not only improve overall health and fitness, but shake things up a bit and break from your routine so it doesn't get tedious.

As with any exercise routine before you plan on adding any kind of cross training activity to your current workout, check with your healthcare professional or personal trainer for its suitability.

CHAPTER 12- PROPER NUTRITION FOR WEIGHTLIFTERS

Nutritional Supplements

You cannot open a weightlifting or muscle magazine without seeing dozens of ads for nutritional supplements. And truth is if you want to bulk up faster and put on weight, supplements can help but it important not to believe all the hype. While nutritional supplementation can help with building muscle, there are no short cuts, and no substitutes for proper training and weightlifting.

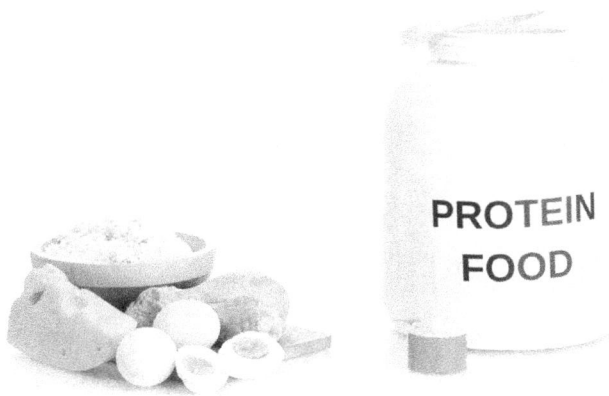

The idea of nutritional supplementation for weightlifting and bodybuilding is a simple one. We know that there is a basic equation to building muscle through weightlifting and resistance training: push your muscles to their limits, followed by appropriate rest to build new muscle, and give your body the proper nutrients it needs to build muscle. Supplementation comes in at that last part of the equation. While many lifters can develop a good routine of "on again/off again" training and can stick to it – always eating the right foods that give the body what it needs to build muscle and build muscle quickly isn't always that easy. Supplements make sure you are giving the body what it needs to recover and build muscle after working out.

Nutritional supplementation for the bodybuilder or weightlifter falls into a few categories, and once again how you supplement will depend on what your ultimate weightlifting goals are. Nutritional supplements for weightlifters are usually products designed to increase muscle like proteins and creatine. Products designed to increase metabolism like fat burners. Supplements that safely simulate the effects of harmful anabolic steroids, and products that aid in recovery and promote joint health like Glucosamine and MSN.

Protein is one of the most essential building blocks to making new muscle. It is cannot be stored in the body so to build muscle you need to constantly replenish your bodies supply of protein. Unfortunately the foods that are highest in protein are often also the highest in fat, and as a bodybuilder or weightlifter you are always trying to decrease your fat intake. Also you are probably loading on carbs, and again most foods high in carbohydrates are low in protein, so most weightlifters will supplement with a good quality protein powder. Protein powders come in variety of types – such as whey protein or soy protein - and flavors, and can be used not only in drinks but in recipes like those found in the Zone diet. Check with your personal trainer or healthcare professional for the right protein supplement for you.

Protein builds muscles, a chemical known as ATP; Adenosine Triphosphate is the fuel that powers them. One of the other most popular supplements that are taken by weightlifters is Creatine. Creatine is naturally found in meat and fish. Creatine when it gets into the muscles combines with phosphate and creates ATP. The more ATP the stronger the muscle and the more resistant it is to fatigue. ATP gives the muscle bursts of energy that allow you to weightlift longer and stronger.

And finally there are the supplements that are the so-called anabolic alternatives. We all know about the dangers of steroids. To avoid the potential problems of taking steroids but to achieve the same type of effect safely, these products all basically work the same way. They use a combination of herbal and other natural ingredients to naturally enhance or stimulate the body's own production of testosterone. And while these products are generally safe, and do not involve the ingesting of hormones, since they are intended to and can change the levels of hormonal activity in the body they should still be used with precaution by teens and women.

Best Protein Powder for Weightlifters

Protein is an essential nutrient for building muscle, and therefore it is an essential part of any weightlifters routine. But protein is not stored in the body, and since it is used to build muscle, the more your build up, the more protein you use, and the more protein you need. It is difficult if not impossible for serious weightlifters to take in all the protein they need to build all that muscle. Most foods that are high in protein are also very high in fat, and as weightlifters or bodybuilders you always want to limit your fat intake. Also most heavy duty lifters have a diet that is high in carbs to bulk up and provide energy – again foods that are high in carbohydrates, are usually low in protein. So most weightlifters will get their protein form shakes made with protein powders.

Protein powder formulations used by weightlifters usually have one of two sources of the protein, soy and Whey. It seems in recent years more weightlifters prefer the Whey protein powders. There has been some evidence that Soy and Soy products limit the production of Testosterone, which is the last thing you want to do as a weightlifter trying to build muscle. Whey protein also has been shown to improve liver function, boost the immune system and act as a natural anti-bacterial and anti-viral.

Whey protein has what is called a very high biological value. Biological value is the amount of protein your body replenishes per 100 grams of ingested protein. If you are interested in protein being used to build muscle, you of course want the highest BV possible. Unlike soy protein, which is derived from a vegetable source, soybeans; whey has a high BV because it derived from milk. "Pound for Pound" or actually in this case "gram for gram" the only source of protein with as high a BV as whey is eggs, but whey does not have the fat or cholesterol component of eggs. Whey protein is also high in essential Amino Acid, which is also important to weightlifters.

Whey protein powders are available from several different manufacturers. Whey protein powders either come unflavored, or can be mixed with any food or juices, or in a verity of flavors to make shakes and drinks. But since it comes from cow's milk in a recent survey many people preferred the taste of even unflavored whey protein over other protein powders, probably because it is derived from milk. Really it becomes matter of personal taste when it comes to choosing any single whey protein powder over another. Any whey protein from any manufacturer is ideal as a weightlifting supplement because it is high quality protein with no fat, no lactose, no cholesterol, is all-natural and is low in calories.

CHAPTER 13- GREAT WEIGHTLIFTING ROUTINES

Weightlifting is no known as great workout for anybody, any sex and just about any age or fitness level. There is not a single human being on the planet above the age of 8 that cannot benefit from reducing fat and building lean muscle mass. That having been said, what then is best weightlifting routine to do that? Take a look at the list I gave you at the start of this paragraph – quite a broad range of people right? And do you think a routine for a 70 year old woman whose weightlifting goal is to increase some strength and fight the effects of osteoporosis – could possibly be the same as a 24 year old competitive bodybuilder? Of course not – the best weightlifting routines are the ones that are best FOR YOU – and for your individual goals.

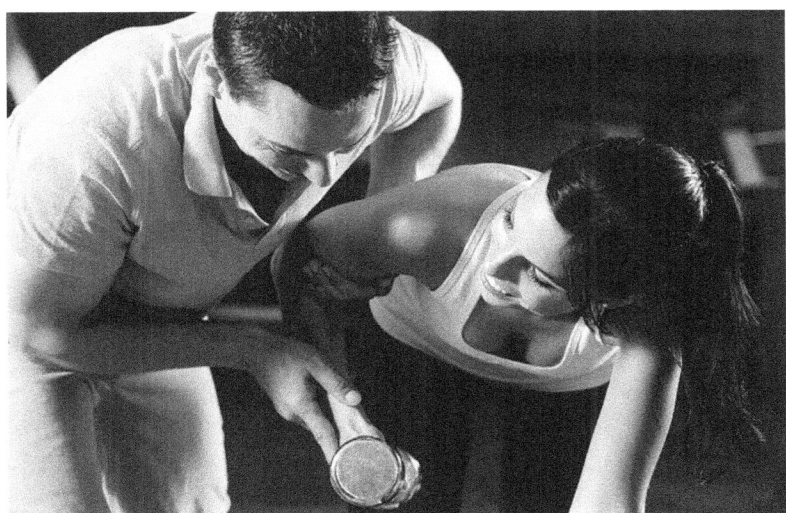

However with that in mind there are some general ideas that all pros agree make any weightlifting goals more achievable. It is always best to clearly define your goals and work with a professional trainer before you begin any weightlifting program. And also check with your doctor, as you should before beginning any exercise regimen.

The basic formula to successfully building lean muscle mass through weightlifting is a simple one.

- Work only one muscle group per day – and be aware of what exercises work multiple muscle groups – a tried and true formula is 5 days on 2 days off.

- Heavy Compound exercises like Squats, Deadlifts etc., work multiple muscle groups and give you more "Bang for your Bucks, so focus on these type of exercises, unless you goal is to build specific muscles for specific sports or daily activities

- Always develop your weekly/daily routine to lift large muscle groups before small one

- Do compound weightlift exercises before isolation exercises

Again the magic of weightlifting as an exercise is that it can be used to improve overall health and physical fitness for your entire life – just ask Jack LaLanne, still pumping at 93! But a weightlifting program also can be targeted and tailor made to work specific muscle groups for specific sports, or even slow the progression of certain disease states like osteoporosis or arthritis. So without getting into specific exercises for your specific goals, experts also recommend the following for getting the most out of a general weightlifting program. Do more compound than isolation exercises, use proper form, and use heavy weights with minimal reps. The key to building muscle is to stimulate muscle growth by pushing muscles to the point of fatigue and stress – heavier weights do this more effectively.

Robert Young

There is a misconception that if you can continue to do rep after rep with a light weight you will get "tone and definition". This is not true. Now that is not to say that doing reps of light weight has no benefit – you are getting a cardio workout doing that – but that is all you are doing – you are doing nothing to build muscle. That is where the familiar term "No Pain – No Gain" comes from. It doesn't mean that weightlifting is supposed to hurt, nor does it refer to the obvious pain you will be in the next day after your first weightlifting session. It means that in order to build muscle, muscle tissue must first be "hurt" it needs to be pushed beyond its limit – so it gets bigger and stronger – it's really is that simple.

CHAPTER 14- Weightlifting-How to be Safe

Weightlifting can be fun. Weightlifting is a great way to get in shape and stay in shape. But like any physical activity weightlifting is not without some inherent risks. The good news is that most of not all of the potentials injuries that can result from weightlifting can be avoided by practicing good technique observing proper safety precautions.

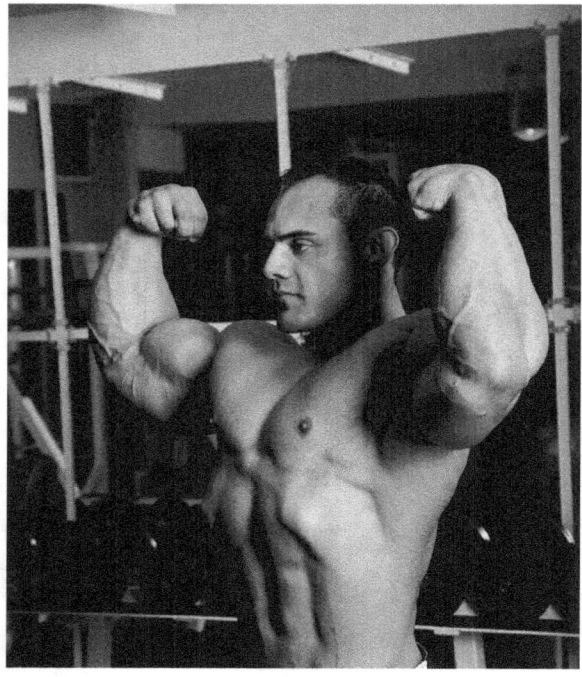

The most common injury related to weightlifting is a back injury. Almost all weightlifting related back injuries occur due to improper technique or lifting beyond ones limitations. Both situations can be easily avoided. If you are prone to a back injury or already have an injured back perhaps you should avoid the weight lifting exercises that are the most common causes of back injury such as Squats or Deadlifts.

For beginners it is far less likely to use improper technique that can result in an injury, by working out on a weight machine, then using free weights. If you do not have the opportunity to be properly trained in the use of free weights, the machines are the way to go. A machine forces you into the right stance or body position for any given weightlifting exercise, and there is little or no possibility of an injury due to a dropped weight while using a machine.

Whether you are weightlifting on a machine or with free weights there are several other weight lifting safety precautions you can take. If you are using free weights, always use a spotter when lifting heavy weights. If no spotter is available be sure to use equipment such as a Squat cage, or press bench that has a place to put the weights on. Weightlifters lifting either with free weights or weight machines should use weightlifting gloves. Gloves ensure a better grip on bars, and prevent blisters and other hand injuries. Wrist straps and wrist hooks can also be used to prevent hand and wrist injuries and add more support to the wrists while working out. Similarly knee braces and back belts can be used where apropos. Weight lifting shoes are a good idea to ensure proper balance and stability when lifting.

Also make sure the equipment is properly functioning. Be sure all pins and clips are secure and in the proper place. Be sure your work out area is free from obstacles and other potential hazards. Do not lift beyond your means, follow a logical progression of slowly increasing the amount of weight or reps. avoid the temptation to "lift to your max". Moderate soreness is OK, and should be expected from ay weightlifting session, however severe pain is not normal. If you are experiencing severe pain stop what you are doing, you are no doubt doing something wrong.

And finally, probably the best way to weightlift safely, ensure proper technique, and avoid injury is to work with a certified personal trainer.

Weightlifting Accessories

Weightlifting is more than just a great way to stay in shape; in fact it is more than just exercise it is a sport. There are both pro and amateur competitive weightlifters, not to mention bodybuilders. And like any sport weightlifting has its share of accessories. Here are some of the essentials.

When we are referring to weightlifting accessories we are talking about anything other than the weights themselves. This can be any piece of equipment or gear that makes the lifting experience easier like weightlifting gloves, to things that help you build up like nutritional supplements. Weightlifting gloves are something that should be worn by any lifter, they prevent blistering and other damage to the hands, and insure a better grip on the weight bars for better form and technique and reduced risk of injury from slippage. Your feet deserve similar protection and there are weight lifting boots. They help provide better balance and a more stable platform for lifting as well as protect the feet from injury. Other types of safety related weightlifting accessories include weight belts and, wrist straps. An ingenious weightlifting accessory in this class is the lifting hook. Lifting hooks have been made to stabilize the wrists and relive stress on hands and wrists while insuring proper bar handling. There are accessories both large and small for specific types of lifting exercises, like weight benches, and head harnesses.

Other accessories include pieces of gear designed to complement or enhance your workouts. Specialized bars fall into this category like curling bars, as do accessories like ankle and wrist weights. A simple yet effective and very popular accessory in this group would be a wrist roller. Basically a dumbbell bar with a cable that you hang a weight plate from and then roll it up. It is probably one of the single most effective ways I know of to strengthen your wrists and forearms, and can be done anywhere.

Then there are other pieces of equipment that are not technically used in actual weightlifting, but are used in complementary exercises that are usually part of a weight-training program. These include, chin up, and pull up bars, push up bars, chest toners, and the ever-popular handgrips and skip ropes. Other weightlifting accessories include those that make your home gym easier to manage and more organized. This would include things like dumbbell racks, plate trees, and other kinds of accessory racks.

Whatever type of weightlifting accessories you are in the market for from a simple set of spring clips for you barbells to a press bench or beyond; there are dozens of discount sites online that sell all sorts of weightlifting accessories at deeply discounted prices.

ABOUT THE AUTHOR

Robert Young was interested in weightlifting from an early age. It was just that his parents though that he was too young to do it. After he started playing football however they relented as he had to do weight training to build muscle and endurance for the games.

It is something that he has not forgotten and he is now the proud owner of a gym in his hometown. He actively participates in his gym also helps to train those who are interested in learning the proper techniques and adhere to the safety precautions of weight lifting. His book is merely way to introduce the individuals that may still be skeptical about weightlifting to what it is all about.

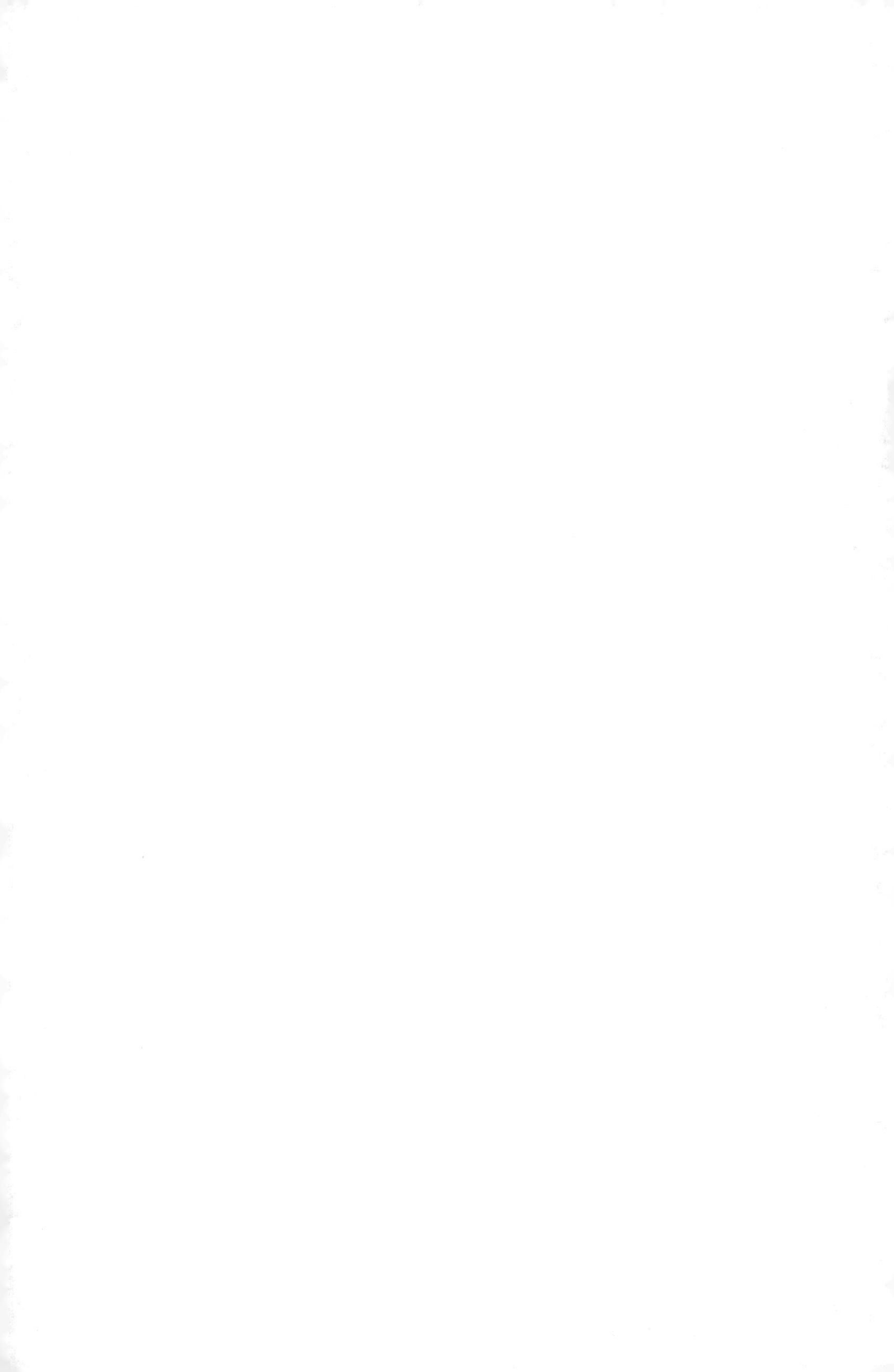

www.ingramcontent.com/pod-product-compliance
Lightning Source LLC
Chambersburg PA
CBHW071122280526
45787CB00003B/1140